A Guide to Ocular Inflammatory Disease

ISBN: 978-0-9994905-2-5

Also available in eBook format

Questions about permission should be addressed to:
Ocular Immunology and Uveitis Foundation
Attn: Alison Justus, Director of Development
PO Box 646 Weston, MA 02451 U.S.A.
E-mail: Ajustus@mersi.com
781-647-1430 x407

Suggested Citation:
Foster, C.S., Foster F.B, Irvin E.A., Manhapra A. (2021)
A Guide to Ocular Inflammatory Disease
The Ocular Immunology and Uveitis Foundation
Weston, Massachusetts

TABLE OF CONTENTS

Anatomy of the Eye

In this drawing, the eye is viewed from the top

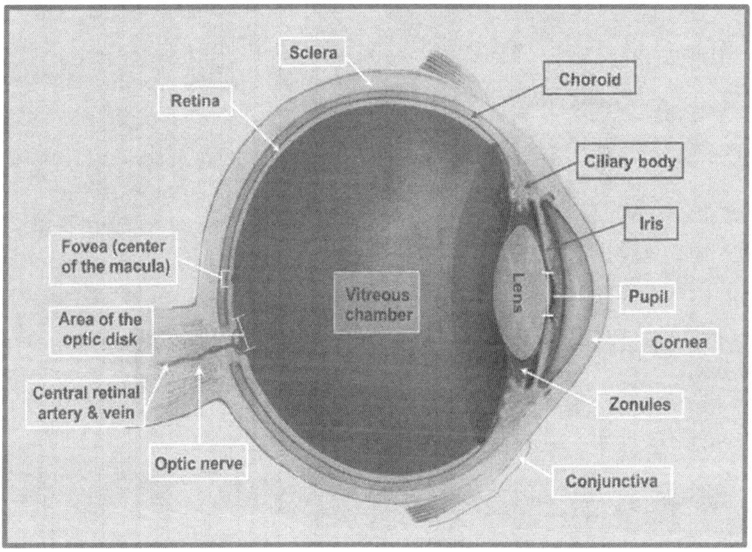

The middle layer of the eye is called the uvea or uveal tract. It is made up of the iris, the ciliary body, and the choroid. The uvea surrounds the eye like a tunic (coat). The visible part of the uvea, in the front, is the iris. Inflammation in any of the parts of the uveal tract is called "uveitis". Inflammation inside the eye is a medical emergency because, untreated, it will lead to vision loss.

To print a diagram of the eye, go to:
http://www.uveitis.org/docs/eye.pdf

Ocular Inflammatory Disease

What is Ocular Inflammatory Disease?

Ocular inflammatory disease is a general term for inflammation affecting any part of the eye or surrounding tissue. Inflammation involving the eye can range from the familiar allergic conjunctivitis of hay fever to rare, potentially blinding conditions such as uveitis, scleritis, episcleritis, optic neuritis, keratitis, orbital pseudotumor, retinal vasculitis, and chronic conjunctivitis.

Broadly speaking, if inflammation develops in the eye(s), or in the optic nerve, blood vessels, muscles or other tissues that surround the eye, the resulting illness is classified as an ocular inflammatory disease (or "OID" for short).

The location of the inflammation governs the diagnostic name for the ocular inflammatory disease. For example, uveitis is inflammation in the uveal tract; scleritis is inflammation of the sclera, pars planitis is inflammation of the pars plana, and so forth.

The Immune System

What is Inflammation?

Literally speaking, inflammation means "setting on fire". Inflammation can develop in any part of the body, including the eyes and their surrounding structures. Inflammation is a characteristic reaction of tissue to injury or disease. Inflammation results from the body's attempt to eliminate a foreign body or germ and helps to prevent further injury.

Inflammation is marked by four signs: swelling, redness, heat, and pain. You have probably observed the signs of inflammation in a cut or burn on your hand.

Inflammation is a complex process involving many different kinds of white blood cells: granulocytes (neutrophils, basophile, and eosoniphils) and some immune specific white blood cells called B and T lymphocytes along with their antibodies and cytokines. In all inflammatory diseases there is the migration of these specific types of white blood cells out of the bloodstream into surrounding tissues. These cells release agents (chemicals), such as cytokines, to boost immune responses and kill invading bacteria, viruses, and parasites or anything that the immune system "perceives" as foreign (antigen), or non-self.

Part of their response is bringing antibodies (proteins in the family of immunoglobulins) to the site; the antibodies then attach to antigens and mark them for death. Antigens are anything that the immune system recognizes as non-self or foreign and, therefore, trigger an immune response. The linking of the antibody to the antigen forms an immune complex. Immune complexes circulate through the blood. Usually they are removed quickly, but occasionally they are lodged into tissues and cause inflammation.

Normal healthy tissue can be injured by inflammation during this process ("innocent bystander injury"). When this happens in or around the eyes, the affected region (the eyes, the eyelids, the sclera, the iris, the uvea, the retina, the optic nerve) becomes red, sore, and swollen. This inflammation can be observed by the eye doctor using a slit lamp microscope. If eye inflammation is long lasting (chronic) or severe, damage to delicate tissues and blood vessels in and around the eye can occur, resulting in vision loss.

Autoimmunity

The immune system is designed to protect and defend the body from foreign intruders (germs). The mechanisms of the immune system reside in the body, not in the eye. The immune system is complex. Essentially, it contains several different types of cells, some of which function like "security guards", which are constantly on patrol looking for any foreign invaders. When they spot one, they take action and eliminate the intruder.

In some forms of ocular inflammatory disease, the immune system loses its ability to tell the difference between a foreign intruder and a person's own normal tissues and cells. So, in essence, the guarding cells lose their memory, and they mistakenly identify the person's own normal cells as foreign (antigens) and, subsequently, take action to eliminate them. This dysregulation of the immune system is termed autoimmunity, or immune attack against self.

The reason why this happens is unknown. The result of autoimmunity is chronic inflammation.

Autoimmune-mediated Ocular Inflammatory Disease (OID)

Autoimmune diseases are characterized by the body's immune responses being directed against its own tissues, causing prolonged inflammation and subsequent tissue destruction. A number of autoimmune diseases exist, the most familiar of which is rheumatoid arthritis. In rheumatoid arthritis, the dysregulated immune system attacks the joints.

A number of autoimmune diseases exist in which the eye or various parts of the eye may be attacked. In ocular inflammatory disease, often the autoimmune disease is systemic, not only involving the eye but a variety of organs throughout the body. The most common examples of such diseases include rheumatoid arthritis, systemic lupus erythematosus, polyarteritis nodosa, relapsing polychondritis, Wegener's granulomatosis, scleroderma, Behcet's disease, inflammatory bowel disease (Crohn's disease and ulcerative colitis), sarcoidosis, and ankylosing spondylitis. Another rare but serious autoimmune condition is thyroid eye disease, also known as Graves' Ophthalmology or Orbitopathy, it is orbital inflammation as a consequence of hyperthyroidism or Graves disease.

Symptoms

However, the eye may in certain instances be the specific and only target affected by certain autoimmune diseases. Some such diseases include ocular cicatricial pemphigoid, Mooren's corneal ulcer, and some forms of uveitis, including Birdshot retinochoroidopathy, Vogt-Koyanagi-Harada syndrome, and sym-pathetic ophthalmia.

What are the signs and symptoms of ocular inflammatory disease?

Inflammation can affect any part of the eye or its surrounding structures. The symptoms of inflammation for the most part depend on the area in the eye of the inflammation. Most common signs and symptoms are:

- Pain
- Redness
- Floaters
- Decreased vision
- Light sensitivity

Eye pain, severe light sensitivity, and any change in vision are considered emergency signs and need immediate attention by an ophthalmologist.

Causes

What Causes Ocular Inflammatory Disease?

The forms of ocular inflammatory diseases that are most commonly seen include ocular allergy, cicatricial pemphigoid, scleritis, peripheral ulcerative keratitis, retinal vasculitis, chronic conjunctivitis, and anterior, intermediate, and posterior uveitis. OID occurs throughout the world. There are over 85 causes of uveitis/OID. They can be infectious or noninfectious, traumatic, drug-induced, or malignant. Both women and men of any race, ethnicity, or age may develop OID.

Infectious causes may be bacteria, parasites, fungus, viruses such as rubella, HIV; sexually transmitted diseases such as syphilis, Chlamydia, or gonorrhea; or rare infections, such as tuberculosis, toxoplasmosis, or Lyme disease.

There are several causes of **noninfectious OID,** one of which is autoimmune disease. In many cases, the autoimmune disease is **systemic** (affecting the body) and, also, produces inflammation in specific parts of the eye. The ocular inflammatory disease will then be identified according to that part of the eye which has inflammation. For example, juvenile rheumatoid (or idiopathic arthritis) is associated with inflammation in the anterior part of the eye, known as anterior uveitis or iritis. The area of inflammation in the eye also is helpful to the doctor in the development of differential diagnoses to detect the cause of your OID.

Autoimmune diseases can also affect just the eye; such as in the following ocular diseases: Birdshot retinochoroidopathy, Fuchs' heterochromic iridocyclitis, Vogt-Koyanagi-Harada, ocular cicatricial pemphigoid. The other cause of noninfectious OID is termed idiopathic. **"Idiopathic" OID** is basically a diagnosis of exclusion. That is, no infection or associated systemic illness can be identified at the time of the diagnosis of eye inflammation. In this instance, inflammation is located entirely in the eye or its structures. This form of OID does not tend to have blood tests that can be used to follow the disease course. The inflammation is evaluated by the doctor using the slit lamp.

Drug or medication can also be the cause of ocular inflammatory disease. Some example drug causes are bisphosphonates, cidofovir, rifabutin, and sulfonamides and latanoprost. Vaccines and even skin tattoos can be inducers of OID. Certain cancers can cause ocular inflammatory disease, such as lymphoma, lung cancer, and breast cancer.

Naming Conventions

Why are there so many names for eye inflammation?

"Itis" is the Greek suffix for inflammation. This suffix is often combined with the name for the part of the eye that has the inflammation to describe the illness.

So, a person may be said to have "iritis" (IRIS + "itis" = I'RI-TIS) when the colored part of the eye (the iris) has inflammation. The term "scleritis" is used, broadly, to describe inflammation of the sclera (SCLER-I'TIS), the tough white outer coat of the eye. "Uveitis" is inflammation of the uveal tract, the middle layer of the eye (U'VE-I'TIS).

Inflammation of the retina will be described as "retinitis". If the vasculature is involved, then it is called "retinal vasculitis". Inflammation in the optic nerve is termed "optic neuritis". Cornea inflammation is "keratitis" and conjunctival inflammation is "conjunctivitis". If both are involved, it is "keratoconjunctivitis"

While this naming convention does not hold true for all inflammatory eye diseases, it helps to explain why there are so many different names for ocular inflammatory disease.

Diagnosis

Getting a Diagnosis

Usually, when an eye problem is suspected, a patient is first sent to a general, comprehensive ophthalmologist. He or she will perform a thorough eye exam, including:

• Tests of visual acuity, to determine if vision has decreased. This can be as simple as reading an eye chart.

• A funduscopic exam, in which the pupil is dilated (widened) so that the ophthalmologist can look into the eye and see structures in the back of the eye.

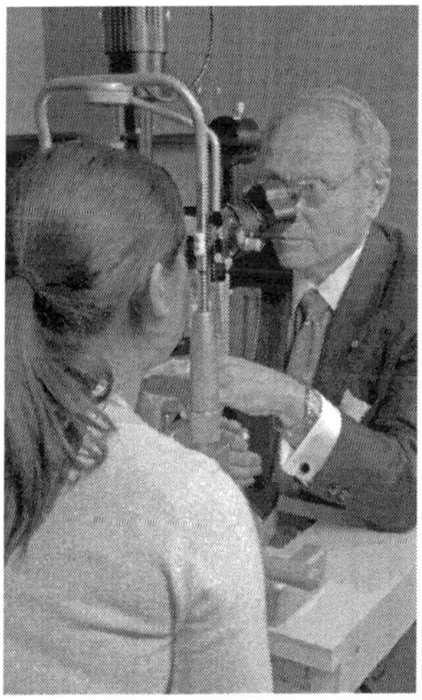

• Measures of the pressure inside the eye to make sure it has not reached levels that might be dangerous. This painless test can be done on the slit lamp by a tonometer or without a slit lamp with a tonometer or a pneumotonometer. These measure the pressure inside the eye by lightly pressing on the surface of the eye.

• A slit lamp exam, in which a narrow beam of light is shone into the eye so that a magnifying lens can closely examine the highlighted portion of the eye.

• Your doctor will use eye drops to dilate the pupil of the eye. A drop of fluorescein dye may also be placed in the eye. This dye temporarily stains the surface of the eye and can help to determine which layers of the eye are inflamed.

• In addition, your physician probably will ask you about your medical history, and will examine you. Depending on the results, he or she may order blood tests and X-rays (such as a chest X-ray to look for evidence of sarcoidosis). Because uveitis often is associated with a viral infection or an autoimmune disease, other conditions need to be discovered and treated as well.

Because ocular inflammatory disease can be caused by so many different things, diagnosis may require a referral to a specialist (an Ocular Immunologist) for further diagnostic evaluation and treatment.

Treatment

The ocular immunologist will review the following, along with his or her exam, to help make the diagnosis:

- The individual's entire medical history
- An analysis of the results obtained in laboratory tests and/or imaging; many times a repeat in serologic testing is needed
- Specialized imaging of the eye and its structures, and
- Some specialized blood tests related to the immune system

How is Ocular Inflammatory Disease Treated?

The treatment of ocular inflammatory disease is aimed at eliminating inflammation. This in return will alleviate pain, stop formation of new floaters, and normalize any acute changes in vision. It is crucial to stop the inflammation before delicate tissues in the eye are damaged in order to prevent secondary complications and permanent vision loss. Our goal of treatment is prevention of recurrence without chronic use of steroids. This goal can be reached by using a treatment stepladder approach explained next.

The Stepladder Approach

The long-term goal is total remission of the ocular inflammatory disease, off of all medication. The road to remission can be bumpy; some forms of ocular inflammatory disease can be very aggressive and "stubborn" to control.

In understanding the treatment of OID, one must remember that the mechanisms of the immune system reside in the body, not in the eye. The treatment of OID is aimed at the cause when it is identifiable. If you have an **infection**, your doctor will prescribe antibiotics or antivirals, etc.

For **noninfectious causes** of inflammation, including idiopathic, treatment will follow a stepladder approach. The object of the stepladder approach is to modify the immune system, to stop it from inappropriately attacking the eye and causing inflammation.

The first step is steroid medication. A steroid is an anti-inflammatory immunosuppressive medication that can be administered in many forms: drops, oral, injection, or intravenous infusion. The form of steroid that is prescribed depends on the severity and type of OID one has. While steroids are effective in quickly aborting acute inflammation, they can result in their own complications if used long term, such as stomach ulcer and osteoporosis.

(bone thinning), diabetes, cataract, glaucoma, cardiovascular disease, weight gain, fluid retention, and Cushing's syndrome.

If inflammation continues to recur after weaning off of steroids, your doctor will move to the next step, nonsteroidal anti-inflammatory drugs (NSAIDS). Some examples of NSAIDS include Motrin, Celebrex, or Naprosyn. NSAIDS are a nonsteroidal type of medication aimed at suppressing inflammation. Oral NSAIDS require monitoring of your liver and kidney function. Certain types of oral NSAIDS, if used long-term, will need added medication for protection against stomach ulcers.

When inflammation persists despite the use of an NSAID, the next step in the stepladder is immunosuppressive chemotherapy medications or immunomodulatory therapy (IMT). These medications include, Methotrexate, CellCept, Imuran, Cyclophosphamide, Leukeran and Cyclosporin plus others. Your doctor will always start with the type that he or she believes is most appropriate for you and your type of OID. In addition, the medication which has the least potential for side effects is favored. The use of such medications requires special, regular monitoring (blood tests) in order to ensure that no hidden side effects are develop. Regrettably, many people (including a surprising number of physicians) are unaware of the very favorable risk-to-benefit ratio of such medications used in the doses that rheumatologists, ocular immunologists, and other specialists prescribe for immunomodulation of autoimmune disease. As a result, many people falsely equate the use of such medications with the high doses given in cancer chemotherapy, with all the risks and side effects that occur at these high doses.

This is not at all what IMT for OID is all about. If used correctly, by a physician who is an expert in such matters, patients with OID who are treated with IMT should look and feel normal. If the patient develops side effects or does not feel good on the IMT, it should be stopped and switched to another IMT. Ultimately, the goal of IMT is to adequately control and stop inflammation in a steroid free manner.

Biologic Response Modifiers

A newer category of medications employed for the treatment of autoimmune diseases called "biologic response modifiers (BRM)" or "biologics" exists. The biologics more specifically target certain elements of the immune system and, in so doing, avoid some of the potential risks of the more conventional IMT medications. Such medications include Humira, Remicade, Acthar, Actemra, Rituximab, intravenous Immunoglobulin (IV-IgG), Orenica, Simponi and others such as Tepezza, approved by the FDA to specifically treat thyroid eye disease, an OID that previously had no approved treatment options.

A BRM medication may be added to a conventional IMT medication in the stepladder approach in aggressiveness of therapy for stubborn inflammation. The efficacy of Humira, one such BRM, was studied by Dr. Foster and other sites using a double masked, placebo controlled, randomized clinical trial and remains the first and only FDA approved biologic that is used to treat non-infectious uveitis. Remicade, another TNF-alpha antagonist, has also been shown to have a favorable influence on ocular inflammation.

It should be noted here that many of the medications mentioned in this pamphlet, including corticosteroids, IMT and BRM medications are not "approved" for treating OID by the United States Food and Drug Administration (FDA). That is to say, the pharmaceutical companies who manufacture these medications have never conducted the randomized clinical trials required by the FDA in order for the companies to include treatment of OID in the package insert or "label" for the medication. Therefore, doctors who employ such medications for treating OID do so "off-label". "Off-label" use is perfectly legal and appropriate, if, in the doctor's opinion, it is in the patient's best interest to proceed with such treatment. One can find in the medical literature many clinical reports in the success of the use of these types of medications mentioned above. For example, Humira was a previously "off-label" medication that is now approved by the FDA for ocular inflammation.

Other medications may also be used in conjunction with immunosuppressants or antibiotics For instance, if inflammation exists in the iris, pupil dilating eye drops may be prescribed to prevent spasms of the muscles of the iris and ciliary body that cause pain. Your doctor may recommend sunglasses because bright light may cause discomfort.

Additional treatment may also be required to treat complications of OID, such as glaucoma and macular edema.

Treatment Duration

Expected Duration of Treatment

The duration of treatment varies person to person and depends on the type and cause of ocular inflammatory disease. Simple forms of uveitis, for example, may respond to treatment within days and may not recur. Chronic (long-term, recurring) forms of ocular inflammatory disease that threaten vision can be very difficult to cure and require persistence on the part of the treating physician(s) and patient. The length of time required to get the disease into a durable remission on IMT is difficult to quantify and is very individualistic, but a minimum of two years is a reasonable estimate. During treatment on IMT, one can expect visits to the ophthalmologist every 4-6 weeks approximately.

With appropriate, targeted treatment, most people with ocular inflammatory disease will become well-controlled and progress to remission. Once in remission from ocular inflammatory disease, you should expect to have regular follow-up visits to your doctor to make sure that the disease remains in remission.

Specialists

What Kind of Doctors Treat OID?

It may be apparent after reading this material that doctors who treat ocular inflammatory disease must have special training in both ophthalmology and in ocular immunology. This type of specialty training is accomplished at an advanced level and is termed Fellowship training. Doctors with this training are specialists in Ocular Immunology, the immunology of the eye, as well as comprehensive ophthalmology. Ocular immunologists, because of their specialty training, are better able to hunt for the cause of your ocular inflammatory disease. Such specialists apply the principles of diagnosis of ocular inflammatory disorders in order to initiate appropriate, disease-directed evaluations. It is the cause of the OID, whether idiopathic or not, that directs treatment. The training of the ocular immunologist also provides him or her with knowledge and experience in the use of the stepladder approach to care. The ocular immunologist is also experienced in knowing when one needs to switch from one IMT to another, how to prevent any potential side effects through close monitoring, and manage side effects if they occur. Furthermore, Ocular Immunologists have special skills with regard to the surgical management of ocular inflammatory disorders.

Support & Coping

Ocular inflammatory disease is a serious illness that affects vision. Because it is a rare illness, you may not know others with your same problem, and you and your family and friends will need to learn about your illness and its treatment.

How people react to serious illness depends on many conditions. Three deserve note. The first is the severity of the illness. Your vision has been affected and you may not feel well in other ways; aggressive medical treatment may be required to save your vision. It is not uncommon to feel distressed in the face of the many decisions that must be made, often quickly. This is quite natural. Ask questions and ask for information.

The second is what social support you have available; if you are willing to ask for help and you have a wide support network, you will have an easier time than if you are isolated. The third condition is your personality; if you have always been pretty resilient, you are likely to have resilience in coping with the illness.

This booklet was developed to provide you with information about your illness. This is an important tool in your recovery. Get informed; learn about your illness. Be a participant in your care.

The Foundation

You and your family may find that you also need support and information in an ongoing way, and the Uveitis/Ocular Inflammatory Disease Support Group offers free services and programs just for you. Ask any staff member about these resources, or look on the website for links (**www.uveitis.org**). Coping with a serious illness such as ocular inflammatory disease means reaching out to others. No question is too small; you are not alone. Consider joining the support group; attend a meeting; get involved! Learn coping skills. It will change your experience with this rare illness.

The Support Group is an educational resource of the Ocular Immunology and Uveitis Foundation (OIUF). The Foundation is the nation's leading 501c(3) non-profit health organization dedicated to:

- Finding cures for ocular inflammatory diseases
- Erasing the worldwide deficit of properly trained ocular immunologists, and
- Providing education and emotional support for those patients afflicted with ocular inflammatory disease.

OIUF is based at the Massachusetts Eye Research and Surgery Institution in Waltham, Massachusetts.

Frequently Asked Questions

Does stress trigger OID?

We do not know definitively in OID, but there is evidence for this in research on a systemic level. There are many anecdotal reports (personal accounts) of patients flaring during or after a stressful time, but this question requires more scientific studies. Although there is no scientific evidence to prove it, we believe that it is possible that certain kinds of stress may play a role in triggering flares of ocular inflammatory disease. Stress does not "cause" the illness itself, but stress is known to modify how the immune system functions. This has implications for stirring up all inflammatory illnesses, including ocular inflammatory disease.

Are flares related to hormones?

Some women notice each time their inflammation flares up, that the episode invariably occurs at the same point in their menstrual cycle, suggesting that certain hormone level changes can be associated with flare ups. It has been noted that OID improves for many during pregnancy. Shanghvi et al postulated that the rapid withdrawal of the anti-inflammatory effects of estrogen and/or progesterone in the late luteal phase may explain the increase in inflammatory attacks during late menstrual cycle. [Menstrual cycle and uveitis. Eye (2004) 18, 451-454].

Are there any medications that people with ocular inflammatory disease should avoid?

There are no absolute contraindications to needed medications for a person with ocular inflammatory disease. Your doctor should watch for allergic reactions to medications. When taking estrogen or oral contraceptives, you should watch for any connections with a change or increase in flare ups. Some medications can cause uveitis as aforementioned in the "causes of OID" section and one should be monitored. There have been no randomized, clinical trials done to date on herbal remedies and treatment of OID. If one is taking medication to suppress the dysregulated immune system, then herbal remedies used to stimulate the immune system would be contraindicated.

Does the Ocular Immunology and Uveitis Foundation conduct research?

Yes. The Foundation is the nation's leading non-profit voluntary health organization dedicated to finding the causes and cure for uveitis and other ocular inflammatory diseases. The majority of support for research comes through tax deductible donations received from patients and other friends of the Foundation. The Foundation is also the recipient of research grants from NIH and industry.

Additional Resources

Other Materials in the Ocular Immunology and Uveitis Foundation Educational Series:

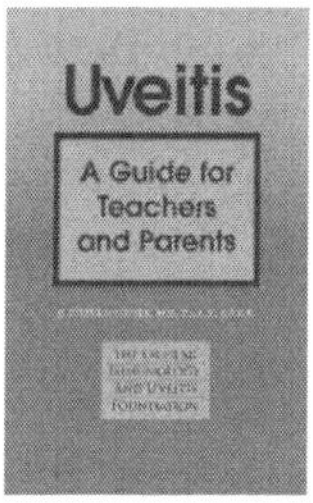

Uveitis: A Guide for Teachers and Parents
C. Stephen Foster, M.D.

Ocular Immunology and Uveitis Foundation. Weston, MA, U.S.A.

Order online:
www.uveitis.org/patients/education/patient-guides

Books by C. Stephen Foster, M.D.

www.uveitis.org/store/category/books

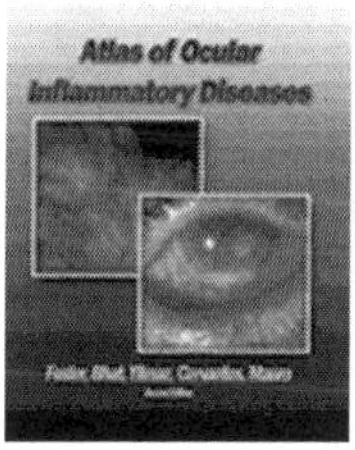

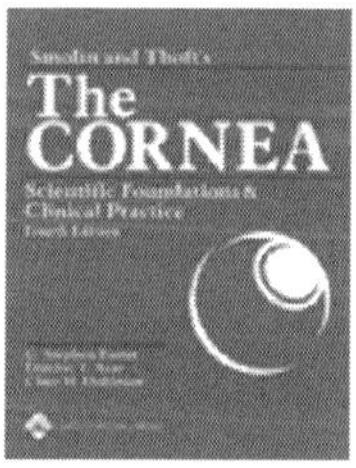

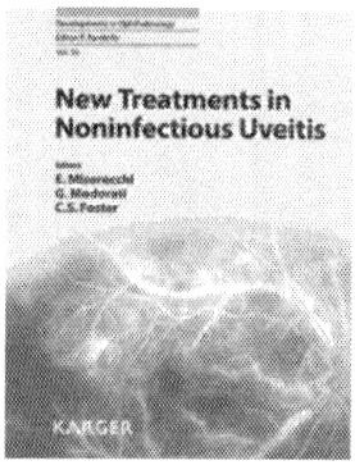

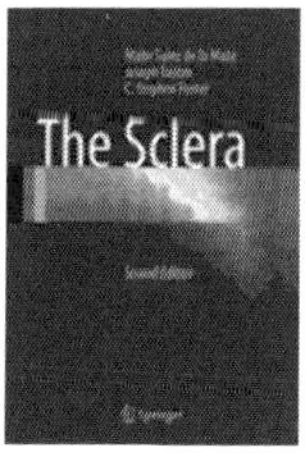

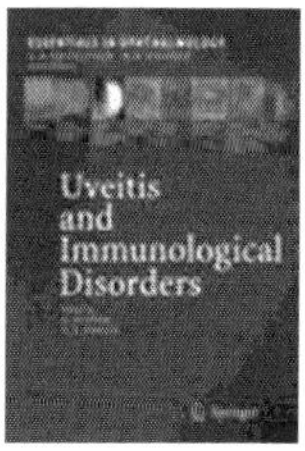

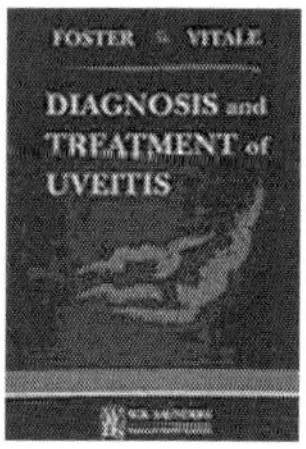

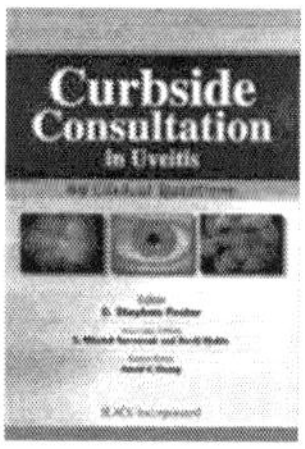

National Eye Institute, National Institutes of Health
Website: www.nei.nih.gov

Foundation Resources

Ocular Immunology and Uveitis Foundation

Massachusetts Eye Research and Surgery Institution (MERSI)
Website: www.Uveitis.org

Glossary of Visions Terms, with Special Reference to Ocular Inflammatory Disease Website:
www.uveitis.org/patients/education/glossary

Resources for Kids and Parents
Website: www.uveitis.org/patients/support/kids

Uveitis/OID Support Group
Website: www.uveitis.org/patients/support

Uveitis Online Support Group, including Group Facebook Page
Website: www.uveitis.org/patients/online-support-group

Links to the OID Treatment Literature
Website: www.uveitis.org/patients/education

Glossary of Terms

Band keratopathy: A deposit of calcium in the cornea. This pathology can be associated with degenerative corneal disease, high blood calcium levels, juvenile uveitis, and chronic uveitis.

Birdshot retinochoroidopathy (BSRC): A chronic intraocular inflammatory disease affecting mainly the back (posterior) part of the eye. BSRC is distinct from other forms of posterior uveitis that have a strong association with the HLA-A29.2 antigen. Its etiology remains unknown. An autoimmune mechanism is likely to play an important pathogenic role.

Blepharitis (anterior blepharitis, posterior blepharitis): An inflammation in the oil glands of the eyelid that results in a chronic or long term inflammation of the eyelids and eyelashes. Symptoms include swollen eyelids and excessive crusting of the eyelashes, most evident in the morning. Tenderness of the eyelids and a foreign body sensation in the eye may occur as well.

Blind spot: Any gap in the visual field corresponding to an area of the retina where no visual cells are present is referred to as a blind spot. There is a naturally occurring blind spot where the optic nerve exists the eye.

Cataract: Protein in the lens of the eye progressively clumps together and clouds the lens, causing a cataract. A cataract can be congenital or develop naturally with aging or can be secondary to chronic inflammation and/or chronic use of steroids.

Cells: The term "cells", as used to in ophthalmology, generally refers to a collection of white blood cells (leukocytes) in the anterior chamber of the eye. Cells can be observed on slit lamp examination floating in the fluid in the front of the eye. The amount of white blood cells is the measure of uveitis activity, and is scaled from 1 to 4, depending on the severity, (1 being the least severe inflammation and 4 being the most severe inflammation).

Inflammatory cells can also accumulate in the vitreous. This occurs as a result of inflammation in intraocular structures such as the ciliary body, retina, and choroid. Cells in the vitreous can be living or dead, and both can become immutably affixed to vitreous fibers. Only live, active cells are graded in the MERSI rating system. Vitreous cells are rated on a scale of 1-4.

Choroid (KOR-oyd): The choroid is a soft, thin, brown, extremely vascular middle layer of tissue that lies between the retina and sclera. It is composed of layers of blood vessels that nourish the back of the eye. Inflammation of the choroids is called choroiditis (KOR-oyd-itis)

Ciliary body: The structure behind the iris responsible for making aqueous humor, the fluid in the front chamber of the eye that nourishes the lens and cornea. The ciliary body is divisible into two parts: the pars plana and the pars plicata anteriorly. The ciliary body is part of the uveal tract. Cyclitis is inflammation of the ciliary body.

Conjunctiva (KAHN-junk-TY-vuh): The conjunctiva is the thin, transparent tissue that covers the outer surface of the eye. It begins at the outer edge of the cornea, covering the visible part of the white part of the eye (the sclera), and lines the inside of the eyelids. The conjunctiva also secretes oils and mucus that moisten and lubricate the eye. Conjunctivitis is an inflammation of the conjunctiva.

Cornea (KOR-nee-uh): The cornea is the outer, transparent, dome-like structure that forms the anterior most part of the outer coat of the eye. Looking through the cornea, as through a window, one can see the iris, pupil, and anterior chamber. The cornea is part of the eye's focusing system. Keratitis is inflammation of the cornea.

Corneal ulcer: See *Keratitis.*

Cyclitis: See Ciliary body

Dry eyes, Keratoconjunctivitis Sicca (KCS): Dry eye syndrome is caused by an alteration in one's natural tear film, a thin layer of tears protecting the surface of our eyes. Damage to the surface of the eyes (cornea and conjunctiva) is responsible for the symptoms of dry eyes which may include irritated, scratchy, dry, uncomfortable or red eyes, a burning sensation or feeling of something foreign in your eyes and blurred vision. Excessive dry eyes may dam- age eye tissue, scar the cornea, and impair vision and make contact lens wear difficult.

Epiretinal membrane (ERM), Macular Pucker: An epiretinal membrane is a thin layer of collagen on the surface of the retina. It may occur spontaneously. It may occur because of inflammation (uveitis), and may occur after vitrectomy. It usually occurs on or near the macula, and therefore affects vision. If it is extremely thin, some call it a "cellophane maculopathy". If it contracts, it distorts the photoreceptors or light-sensing neural elements of the macula, producing "macular pucker".

Episcleritis: *See Sclera*

Eyelids: The eyelids are composed of an outer layer of skin, a middle layer of muscle and tissue that gives them form, and the inner layer of conjunctiva. The eyelids play a key role in protecting the eye's surface by spreading moisture (tears) over the surface of the eyes through blinking.

Flare: Flare is protein in the anterior chamber caused by leakage from inflamed blood vessels in the iris. It is not always a measure of inflammation. Flare is measured on a scale from 1 to 4, with 4 being the most severe. Flare becomes chronic after inflammation has produced permanent changes to blood vessels, and so "flare" may be present even when the patient is not having a "flare-up" of inflammation. Flare in the vitreous can also be observed and rated.

Floaters: Floaters appear as gray or black specks, strands, or "cobwebs" in front of the eyes. As thc eyes move, the floaters move too. Floaters are caused by particles, such as white blood cells and vitreous condensates, suspended in the vitreous gel, the clear, jelly-like fluid that fills the inside of the eye. The floaters cast shadows on the light sensitive retina. It is actually the shadow of the floater that you see.

Fuchs' heterochromic iridocyclitis: A chronic, unilateral anterior uveitis characterized by iris heterochromia, a condition in which one eye is a different color from the other. The uveitis typically occurs in the lighter colored eye of a young adult.

Glaucoma: Glaucoma is a condition characterized by vision loss due to irreversible damage to the retina and optic nerve from an imbalance between the blood flow and the pressure in the eye. In most instances, this imbalance of forces occurs as a result of pressure in the eye that is too high. Although normal pressure is usually between 12-21 mm Hg, a person might have glaucoma even if the pressure is in this range.

HLA-B27 associated uveitis: HLA-B27-associated uveitis occurs, we think, as a result of some germ or other triggering an autoimmune response. Certain germs have proteins that "look" like part of the HLA-B27 protein that is present on the surface of the cells of the body in patients who inherit the HLA-B27 gene. And if such a person has the bad luck to come into contact with one of those certain germs at some point in life, the person's immune system will, of course, attack and kill the germ; but it may also then inappropriately begin to "see" part of the HLA-B27 protein as also being foreign or germ-like, and attack it too, producing damage to the patient's own cells

Idiopathic: When the ocular inflammatory disease cannot be associated, at the time of evaluation, with a particular systemic illness, it is said to "idiopathic".

Intraocular pressure (IOP): A measure of the pressure inside the eye; normal IOP varies among individuals. Intraocular pressure is measured using a tonometer.

Iris: The iris is the most anterior part of the uvea. It is the colored ring of tissue suspended behind the cornea and immediately in front of the lens. It regulates the amount of light entering the eye by adjusting the size of the pupil. When we say that someone has "green, or brown, or "blue" eyes, we are describing the color of the iris. Iritis is inflammation predominantly located in the iris.

Iridocyclitis: A term used to denote inflammation in two parts of the uveal tract of the eye; the iris and the ciliary body

Keratitis, peripheral ulcerative Keratitis: Keratitis is inflammation of the cornea, the outer, transparent, dome- like structure that forms the anterior most part of the outer coat of the eye. If ulcers develop in the peripheral cornea, it is referred to as peripheral ulcerative Keratitis.

Keratic precipitates (KP): Clumps of white blood cells deposited onto the back of the cornea.

Lacrimal gland (LAK-rih-mul): The small almond-shaped structure that produces tears; located just above the outer corner of the eye, behind the eye lid.

Lens: The transparent, double convex (outward curve on both sides) structure suspended between the aqueous and vitreous. It is part of the eye's focusing system. The lens is made mostly of water and protein. The protein is arranged to let light pass through and focus on the retina.

Macula (MAK-yoo-luh), Fovea: The macula is located roughly in the center of the retina, temporal to the optic nerve. It is a small and highly sensitive part of the retina responsible for detailed central vision. The fovea is the very center of the macula that provides the sharpest vision.

Macular edema, Cystoid Macular Edema (CME): When the macula accumulates fluid, it tends to swell like a sponge. This swelling occurs in tiny grape-like clusters and looks like a cyst, hence the name cystoid macular edema (CME). CME can cause permanent loss of central vision if not properly treated.

Multifocal choroiditis and Panuveitis: Multifocal choroiditis and panuveitis (MCP) is a posterior chorioretinal inflammatory disease of unknown etiology with prominent elements of vitritis and anterior segment uveitis. MCP is more often resistant to treatment with systemic and regional steroids. Immunosuppressive treatment has been found to be effective.

Neovascularization: In proliferative retinopathy, new, fragile blood vessels grow on the surface of the retina and on the optic nerve. These new blood vessels are called neovascularization, and can lead to serious vision problems, because the new vessels can break and bleed into the vitreous. In addition, abnormal blood vessels can grow on the iris, which can lead to glaucoma

Ocular allergy: The terms "ocular allergy" and "allergic conjunctivitis" are used synonymously because the large majority of eye allergies involve the conjunctiva. The clinical presentation of the various forms of allergic conjunctivitis can be mild to severe with vision-threatening complications.

Ocular cicatricial pemphigoid (OCP): A systemic autoimmune disease. Mounting evidence supports the concept of immunoregulatory dysfunction: antibodies are directed against the basement membrane zone (BMZ) of the conjunctiva and other mucous membranes derived from stratified squamous epithelia and occasionally the skin. OCP is a vision threatening illness that usually requires treatment with immunosuppression.

Optic nerve, optic disc, optic nerve head: The circular area (disc) where the optic nerve connects to the retina. The brain receives information from the optic nerves for the left visual field and the right visual field. Optic neuritis is inflammation of the optic nerve.

Pars plana: The pars plana is part of the ciliary body. The ciliary body is divisible into two parts: the pars plana and the pars plicata anteriorly. Pars planitis is inflammation of the pars plana, a part of the ciliary body. Pars planitis is one form of intermediate uveitis where some physicians may use the term intermediate uveitis, instead of pars planitis.

Peripheral Vision (per-IF-ur-al): Side vision. The ability to see objects and movement outside of the direct line of vision.

Pupil: The pupil is the adjustable opening at the center of the iris that allows varying amounts of light to enter the eye. The pupil appears dark because the inside of the eye has no light.

Retina: The retina is the light-sensitive layer of nerve tissue that lines the rear two-thirds of the eye. The retina converts images from the eye's optical system into electrical impulses sent along the optic nerve to the brain. The retina contains one million photoreceptors that capture light rays and convert them into electrical impulses. These impulses travel along the optic nerve to the brain where they are turned into images. There are two types of photoreceptors in the retina: rods and cones. Retinitis is inflammation of the retina. See UVEITIS; POSTERIOR UVEITIS.

Retinochoroidopathy: Pathology or abnormality of retina and choroids.

Sclera (SKLEH-ruh): The tough, white, outer layer (coat) of the eyeball made up of connective tissue fibers. With the cornea, it forms the outer wall or coat of the entire eyeball. Six tiny muscles connect to the sclera around the eye and control the eye's movements. The optic nerve penetrates the sclera at the very back of the eye. The sclera is covered by the episclera, a thin layer of tissue containing many blood vessels that nourish the sclera. At the front of the eye, the episclera is covered by the conjunctiva. Episcleritis, inflammation of the episclera, is usually mild and rarely progresses to scleritis, inflammation of the sclera.

Superficial punctate Keratitis: A condition in which cells on the surface of the cornea are inflamed. The cause may be a viral infection, a bacterial infection, dry eyes, exposure to ultraviolet light (sunlight, sunlamps, or welding arcs), irritation from prolonged use of contact lenses, or irritation from or an allergy to eye drops. The condition can also be a side effect of certain drugs taken internally, such as vidarabine.

Synechiae (SIN-eeky-eye): Adhesions of the iris to the lens (posterior synechiae) or to the back of the corneal periphery (peripheral anterior synechiae). Focal adhesions will result in an irregularly shaped pupil and may produce secondary angle closure glaucoma due to relative pupillary block.

Tears: The function of tears is to bathe, lubricate, and nourish the surface of the eye. Tears also contain antibodies that help protect the eye from infection. Tears are produced by the lacrimal (tear) glands, located near the outer corner of the eye. The fluid flows over the eye and exits through two small openings in the eyelids (lacrimal ducts); these openings lead to the nasolacrimal duct, a channel that empties into the nose.

Trabecular meshwork (truh-BEC-yoo-lur): The trabecular meshwork is the spongy, mesh-like tissue surrounding the iris that allows the aqueous fluid (humor) to flow to Schlemm's canal then out of the eye through ocular veins. See Glaucoma.

Uvea (Uveal tract) (YOO-vee-uh): The uvea (from the Latin, uva or grape) is composed of iris, ciliary body, and choroid. Each of these components of the uvea has a unique histology, anatomy, and function. The choroid is the intermediate of the three coats of the eyeball, sandwiched between the sclera and the retina. Anteriorly, the iris controls the amount of light that reaches the retina, whereas the ciliary body is responsible for aqueous humor production.

Uveitis: Uveitis is inflammation inside the eye, specifically affecting one or more of the three parts of the eye that make up the uvea: the iris (the colored part of the eye), the ciliary body (behind the iris, responsible for manufacturing the fluid inside the eye) and the choroid (the vascular lining tissue underneath the retina). Uveitis is the third leading cause of blindness in the developed world.

Anterior uveitis: Inflammation in the front (anterior) part of the eye, in the area between the cornea and the iris. This inflammation derives primarily from inflammation of the iris.

Intermediate uveitis: A term used to denote an idiopathic inflammatory syndrome mainly involving the anterior vitreous, peripheral retina, and ciliary body, with minimal or no anterior segment or chorioretinal inflammatory signs.

Posterior uveitis: Inflammation predominately located in the posterior vitreous, retina, and/or choroid. Posterior means "rear" or "back". Posterior uveitis is a vision disorder characterized by inflammation of the layer of blood vessels underlying the retina, and usually of the retina as well.

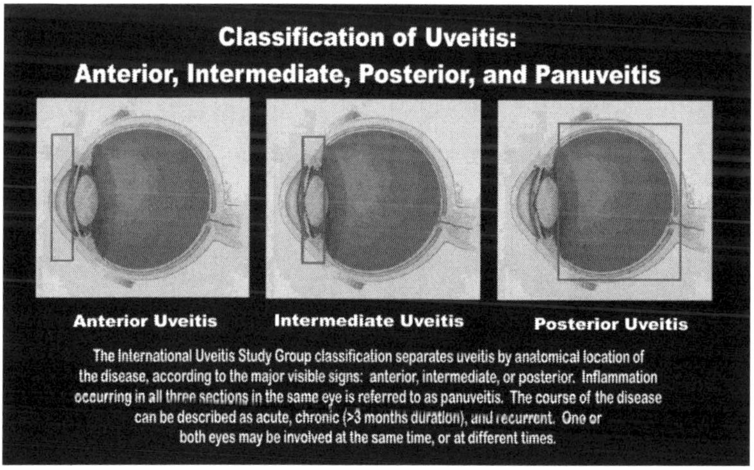

Panuveitis: When inflammation is located in multiple parts of the same eye (anterior, intermediate, and posterior sections), it is classified as panuveitis.

Vasculitis: Vasculitis is inflammation in the blood vessels. It may occur throughout the body. When inflammation occurs in the blood vessels of the retina, it is referred to as retinal vasculitis.

Vitreous (VIT-ree-us): The transparent, colorless, that fills the space between the lens of the eye and the retina lining the back of the eye. It contains very few cells, no blood vessels, and 99% of its volume is water. Unlike the fluid in the front of the eye (aqueous fluid) which is continuously replenished, the gel in the vitreous chamber is stagnant. Therefore, if cells or other byproducts of inflammation get into the vitreous, they will remain there unless removed surgically with a vitrectomy.

Vogt-Koyanagi Harada (VKH): Vogt-Koyanagi-Harada syndrome (VKH), formerly known as uveomenigitic syndrome is a systemic disorder involving multiple organ systems, including the ocular, auditory, nervous, and integumentary (skin) systems. Severe bilateral panuveitis associated with subretinal fluid accumulation is the hallmark of ocular VKH.

Zonules: The fibers that hold the lens suspended in position and enable it to change shape during accommodation. Zonules attach to the ciliary body.

Uveitis/OID Support Group Fund

Ocular Immunology and Uveitis Foundation

Contributions from people like you helped pay for the printing of this booklet. If you would like to help sustain this important work, please consider a tax deductible donation to the Uveitis/OID Support Group Fund.

Make your check payable to the:
Ocular Immunology and Uveitis Foundation

Please complete and include this card so we know where to direct your donation, and mail to:
PO Box 646' Weston, MA 02493 U.S.A.

Your name:______________________________

Address:______________________________

____

Phone
or email:______________________________

Donations to the Foundation are tax deductible. 100% of your directed donation to the Uveitis/OID Support Group Fund goes to support our free educational and support programs.

$

Amount enclosed

THE OCULAR IMMUNOLOGY AND UVEITIS FOUNDATION

A Guide to Ocular Inflammatory Disease

Please direct inquiries or comments to:

Alison Justus
Director of Development and Programs
Ocular Immunology and Uveitis Foundation
PO Box 646 Weston, MA 02493
E-mail:ajustus@oiuf.org
781-647-1431 ext 407

Connect with us!

www.twitter.com/uveitis1/

www.facebook.com/ocularimmunologyanduveitisfoundation

www.instagram.com/oiuf2020/

www.linkedin.com/company/the-ocular-immunology-and-uveitis-foundation

Made in the USA
Monee, IL
19 May 2026

50510984R00026